SWEET SAVASANA

SURRENDERING TO STILLNESS

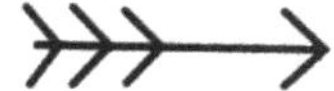

COURTNEY CLAPPER

Edited by
ALEXANDRA CAMPBELL

To all the overworked, overspent, underloved, and underslept …

Shut up.
Lie down.
Breathe in.
Breathe out.

…especially if you do not have time

शवासन

SAVASANA | SHAVASANA

Pronounced: Shah-vahs-uh-nuh
Defined: Final Relaxation Pose/Final Resting Pose

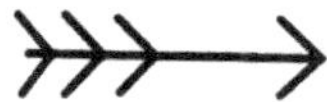

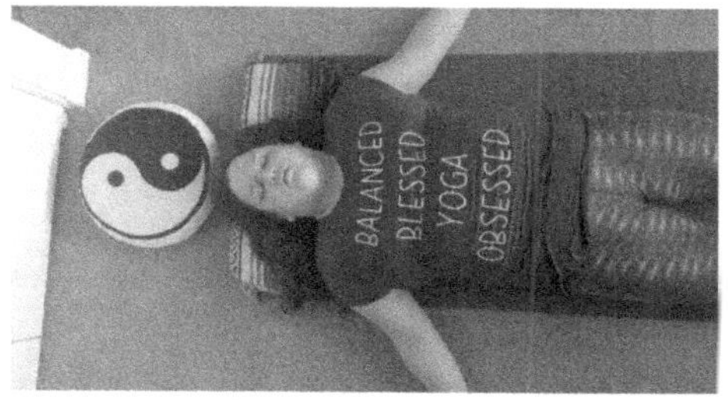

As you come to the end of a yoga class, the teacher will gener-
ally bring you to complete stillness.

You simply
    (but not so simply)
        lie on your back,
            flat on the floor,
                palms faced up,
                    creating space
                        every inhale,
                            releasing further
                                every exhale.

Resting. In. Peace.

It is a wonderful way to wind down class while allowing the body to fully soak in all the benefits of yoga asana.

In Savasana, the body is in (what is suppose to be) the most optimal aligned position for resting.

The entire body is fully supported equally, making it able to relax completely--if you let yourself relax.

In this optimal resting state, you may lie there simply focusing on the breath, or if you are in a class, you may be lead by the instructor on where to place your attention.

Savasana lead in a yoga class can go in so many different directions, working on different areas and aspects of the body, from: focusing on the breath going into a body scan, in which you are bringing awareness to each body part ending with total awareness and relaxation of the body; going into a chakra scan, in which you may be lead to invision colors, maybe flowers, as you work your way through opening, balancing/activating and closing the chakra system; or even, going into being walked through some delightful visual scene, often a journey of some sort (maybe leading your relaxed mind into your subconscious).

This is what you are instructed to do.

There is so much more that happens underneath the surface while we are in this pose.

Savasana is truly the "final resting pose".

You are learning to let go of everything.

Translated to Corpse Pose, whether you are consciously aware of it or not, you are learning to literally let go of every-thing.This is the position in which you are to die a peaceful death---and this is a friendly reminder that, we are all going to die.

You are releasing all your worries, your tension, your need to be busy, your need to be in control, your expectations, and most importantly, you are releasing what no longer serves the better good for yourself.

Similar to meditation, your mind may wander. This is just the nature of the mind...it creates thoughts.

Once you notice you are not with your breath in your body, but in your mind with your thoughts...know your attention has already made way back to your breath, by that simple act of noticing; continue with this cycle.

This is why, it may actually be the toughest pose of all.

Can you let go?

Can you release?

Can you be still?

Can you turn in and tune in?

Can you relax without falling asleep?

Can you just lie down and simply be?

Referencing my Kula Kamala YTT Manual, Mind Body Connection & Stress:

> Because our bodies respond to what we think, feel and do, when we are stressed, anxious or upset physically, mentally and/or emotionally, our body takes on a level of dis-ease, which when unaddressed for some time manifests as or contributes to deeper and more permanent forms of disease.
>
> The Sympathetic Nervous System responses increase during stressful breathing. While your SNS is stimulated your muscle tension, heart rate, perspiration and mental agitation increases, while blood clotting and intestinal function decrease because you are impairing your optimal breathing patterns.

When you fully relax in Savasana, the body becomes at ease, the breathing becomes absolutely natural, and you are simply being (a human being).

Your entire being returns to a balanced state on all levels; physically, mentally, emotionally, and spiritually.

The object is actually allowing yourself to relax and get into a state of homeostasis; which is defined as *the tendency toward a relatively stable equilibrium between interdependent elements, especially as maintained by physiological processes.*

As well as, doing your best at maintaining that state after coming out of the practice, all the while, practicing more to make that state a more common occurrence within your being.

SOME SAVASANA TIPS

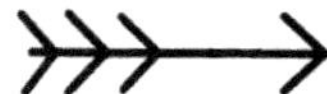

- Your body will wind down much easier for you if you exercise right before...even if maybe you are practicing at night before bed...do a round or two of Surya Namaskar, Sun Salutation, or even more suitable, Chandra Namaskar, Moon Salutation, (especially if you suffer from insomnia on any level), then do Savasana to let yourself completely relax. This may help if you have trouble sleeping. You can even do this lying in bed, covered up, nice and cozy; you may just fall right to sleep, mid-savasana.

- If you like to use essential oils, feel free to use your favorite relaxation blend. Same with crystals. Make it a fun practice for yourself.

- I personally LOVE and ALWAYS try to do one final "Breath of Release" I say, or cleansing breath; inhaling as deep as you can through your nose and

exhaling fully and completely in one big sigh though
your mouth (maybe two or three times, as much as
needed)

- Scan, notice and relax your entire body. This allows
  you to relax areas that you may keep engaged without
  realizing: i.e. the glutes, the shoulders or maybe
  the jaw.

- Hold true gratitude for yourself for giving you the
  time to just focus on you, in your being.

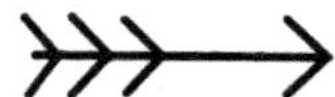

- Ideally, you are to be lying flat on the floor, no props, completely aligned.

- Like myself, if you feel you are decreasing space between the back of your head and the top of your spine, place a folded blanket or pillow under your head, just to where your cervical spine (your head and neck) is in line with your thoracic spine (your back); your gaze will be straight in front of you.

- For lower back or knee pain, place a rolled blanket under your knees, just to raise them up, allowing your lower back to rest.

- Feel as though your eyes never stop fluttering? Invest in, or maybe DIY your very own eye mask/pillow. Possibly, also relaxing your face muscles.

- Anxiety? Look into getting one, or some, sandbag(s);
  one can be placed on your lower belly (pelvic area),
  with two, you can place one in each palm. Sometimes,
  having the extra weight to melt into the floor
  can help.

- Get chilly? Get a blanket and tuck yourself in,
  with love.

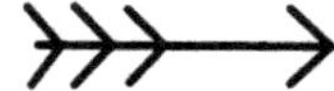

- How often you do simply let yourself relax? Savasana!

- How much time do you practice your concentration/focus/awareness/consciousness? Take the time in Savasana.

- When do you actually let yourself observe you, your life, your mind, your body, your feelings, your thoughts, your world, without any judgement? Observe all of this during Savasana.

- Sore muscles? Let them relax in Savasana.

- High blood pressure? Anxiety? Insomnia? See if you may find relief with Savasana.

- Want to get to know yourself on a deeper level? Dive in through Savasana.

SCIENCE OF SAVASANA

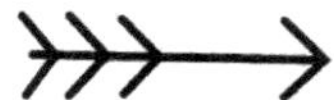

MAJORITY of us are able to be aware of what is going on to the outside of our body; we learn at a very young age where our mouth is in order to be able to feed ourselves when hungry. Also, involving knowing where our arms and hands are in time and space to grab said food. This is called *proprioception*. (We are pretty brilliant organisms)

We also have a counter-sense allowing us to be aware of what is going on in our inside body. I found a fantastic piece on the concept of *interoception* during a Savasana practice in an article on www.doyouyoga.com "The Holistic Benefits of Savasana":

> Practice will increase body awareness and interoception. Interoception is insight on the physiological condition of the body and is associated with the autonomic nervous system and autonomic motor control. The autonomic nervous

system is in control of the normally unconscious and automatic bodily functions like breathing, the heartbeat, and the digestive processes.

Interoception is also linked to the formation of subjective feeling states. In summary, practicing Savasana may increase the ability to notice things like the body's breathing and heartbeat as well as form calmer and more relaxed feeling states.

For this reason, increased interoception has been linked to decreased signs and symptoms of anxiety and depression. In addition, savasana is known as a great way to calm the mind, reduce stress and fatigue, lower blood pressure, relieve headache pain, and improve sleep.

By gaining more connection with being able to be aware of and access our inner worlds, we are able to learn and listen to what our body truly needs to live healthy. Whether that be taking a couple extra minutes in your Savasana relaxation, or maybe understanding that you do need to get a little exercise in beforehand to really release your excess energy.

This is all about building a better relationship with yourself, so you can better serve yourself. You learn more about how your inner body physically, mentally and emotionally functions and then learn ways to make the movements that may be tough for you now, less and less troublesome (physically, mentally and emotionally) as you continue with your practice; taking things just one Savasana at a time.

WORK CITED

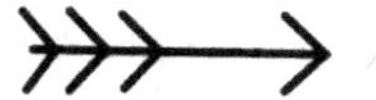

Allitt, Sudha. *Kula Kamala Foundation 200 YTT Manual.* Reading: Kula Kamala Foundation, 2007. Print.

Beisecker, Ling. *The Holistic Benefits of Savasana.* DoYouYoga.-com. <https://www.doyouyoga.com/the-holistic-benefits-of-savasana-57950/> Accessed 19 September 2018.

A SAVASANA POEM

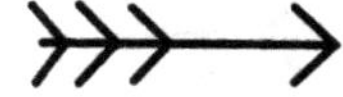

Lying there, steady.
Doing nothing, only
On the outside.

*inhale "I know I am breathing in"
*exhale "I know I am breathing out"

Only on the inside
Am I working.
So vast. So complex, yet simple.

* inhale "I know I am breathing in"
*exhale "I know I am breathing out"

Feet; toes, soles, tops.
Ankles, calves, knees.
Thighs, hips, glutes.
Lower back, upper back.
Shoulder blades.
Lower belly, upper belly.
Chest.
Heart.
Hands; fingers, palms, backs.
Wrists, forearms, elbows.
Upper arms, shoulders.
Neck, sides of neck.
Jaw, cheeks, temples, lips, tongue,
mouth.
Nose, ears.
Eyes, eyebrows.
Forehead, sides of head.
Crown of head.
Whole body relaxing.

*inhale "I know I am breathing in"
*exhale "I know I am breathing out"

Whole body relaxing.
Lower body, upper body.

Whole body relaxing.
Mind relaxing.

Inhale. Exhale.
Breathe in. Breathe out.
Take in. Give out.

Paradox, relax.

~Paradox, relax.

September 19, 2018
Courtney Clapper

THE BREATH: A SHORT SAVASANA VIDEO

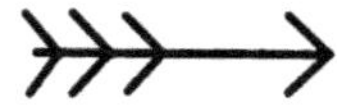

https://youtu.be/31QXZp3pntg

PLEASE WATCH and use the video along with this book for more of a visual reference of the pose, props, and a short savasana meditation at the end.

...a little something extra, just for you (: Hope you enjoy!

A SPECIAL THANKS

First, I want to thank my yoga school, Kula Kamala Foundation and Ashram; Sudha, Ed and everyone involved. My time there taught me so much and left me with such beautiful memories. For more information, please visit: www.kulakamalafoundation.org

My teacher training also allowed me to meet the very person that blessed me with her amazing editing skills and knowledge for this very book, Alexandra Campbell; teaching me something new about words and writing almost every time we talk.

I would also like to thank every single yoga teacher who has brought me into Savasana; each one always a little different, but never fails to be so restoring.

Of course, I obviously cannot leave out you, my reader: much appreciation for you taking the time to learn more about the (easy, but not so easy) amazing practice and pose of Savasana, and what it means to me.

Lastly, I want to give a very special thanks to my own mind and body, for letting me experience this beautifully refreshing rest in silence and stillness.

ABOUT THE AUTHOR AND BOOK

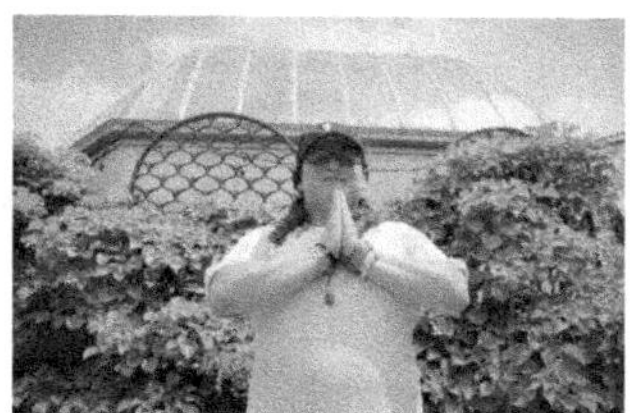

My name is Courtney Clapper, I graduated as a 200CYT in May 2018 from Kula Kamala, and have been practicing yoga as a student since 2007.

I am fascinated with Svadhyaya, or self-study.

I love to practice and teach everything involving slowing down the breathe, the flow, the body, the mind, the entirety of the moment---and just noticing.

Mainly, because I feel it is what we do least in our go-go-go society; most of the time, always feeling the need to have to be doing something to be productive, and if we are not busy doing something, we are being lazy--this is NOT always the case.

A lot can be noticed when you slow things down, allowing you the time to actually pay attention to things you may have not before. And speaking of Savasana specifically, a lot can happen when you are "doing nothing."

I, hopefully, provided you a bit of information, you find valuable for yourself, about Savasana (obviously), along with yoga, and maybe even your own mind and body.

To read more about me and what I teach: www.doyogabelove.wordpress.com

Now please, go, shut up, lie down, breathe in, and breathe out.

So much love for you! Namaste ॐ

facebook.com/doyogabelove

twitter.com/doyogabelove

instagram.com/courtneydocourtneybe